GOD'S LOVE IS SERIOUS

Winning the War Against Cancer

by
Merrily Opal Pearl

Editor – Ashley Kellis

GOD'S LOVE IS SERIOUS
WINNING THE WAR AGAINST CANCER

Published through Firewalker Publishing
www.firewalkerpublishing.com

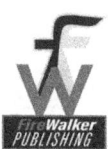

All rights reserved
Copyright © 2022 by Merrily Opal Pearl
Cover art copyright © 2022 by Firewalker Publishing

ISBN: 978-0-9892719-1-2 (Paperback Edition)
ISBN: 978-0-9892719-2-9 (eBook Edition)

No part of this publication may be reproduced, stored in a retrieval system, or transmitted in any form or by any means electronic, mechanical, photocopying, recording, or otherwise, without the written permission of the author or publisher.

Bible Quotations from: The Holy Bible,
New International Version 1990

Some names have been changed in this book
to protect and to be protected.

Dedication/Acknowledgements

This book is dedicated to God, who keeps me here and gives me my purpose—helping others. God is first. Without Him, I would not exist.

My life has been greatly enriched and influenced by my family, friends, doctors, pastors, neighbors, teachers, and children. I am grateful for all who took part in helping this book become a reality. Each one of you has shaped my life in unique and different ways. God blesses us with each other, and I appreciate what each of you has given to me in my life's journey.

Finally, I would like to acknowledge Ernest W. Phillips. God gave me a task: to be a helper to someone who was going to be a great and mighty helper of man. Ernest W. Phillips is the single most influential person on this Earth. He has helped me be a better person, and I am honored to use the talents God has given me to be of assistance to him.

God honors faith, and faith honors God.

II Samuel 22:33
It is God who arms me with strength and makes my way perfect.

Psalm 28:7
The Lord is my strength and my shield; my heart trusts in him, and I am helped. My heart leaps for joy and I will give thanks to him in song.

INTRODUCTION

I have written this to help people going through a difficult time with health issues. I have lived with health issues all my life, and in my fifties, I was given the diagnosis of cancer. God has always been there to lean on. God can make a way where there is no way. This book is meant to be a testimony that you can win the war against cancer with God's help.

I am a survivor. A survivor is someone, or something, that remains here alive and intact. They outlived, or outlasted, the disaster or circumstances in which they found themselves. Surviving is for a period of time. To go beyond this point, to take what comes and make a change, is to be one who thrives. I am a thriver, and I share this with others. I want more people to thrive. We each have a purpose in life that God has given to us. May God give you the courage to push toward the purpose you are given.

God has been my helper in keeping me here and in writing this book. God has sent people into my life to help me with lessons I have needed to learn. I am grateful to all the people who helped me become a better person. I am blessed to be a miracle of the living God and to have the chance to share my life story with others here on Earth.

The medical field has made leaps and bounds into multiple treatment options to extend and save lives. Ask God for guidance through this difficult time, and lean on Him with your decisions.

When peace from God takes away the fear, you know you have made the choice that is right for you.

    I understand that battles and skirmishes can be lost, but the war God fights is always won in the end. Death is but a doorway to a better place. Life is a gift to share the lessons you have learned. God wants us to share with others, so people can be encouraged to fight on and have hope for the future.

Psalm 34:7
The angel of the Lord encamps around those
who fear him, and he delivers them.

Psalm 48:14
For this God is our God for ever and ever;
he will be our guide even to the end.

Chapter One

Begin with God

Beginnings are something fresh and exciting. They bring about strong feelings within each of us. We may have mixed emotions—excitement that something new is coming and the worry that we may not be ready for it.

How many times do we go through a beginning? Each moment has the potential to be a wrapped and bottled new beginning.

God made time. He was here before time and will be here long after time has ended. Some say there are great moments in time. But I believe there is more to the story. Every moment has a moment before this moment right now and the one that follows. You cannot pluck one out and say it is greater than another. God made it so each moment interconnects, so they intertwine and interlock, becoming stronger from the moment before. To build the big picture, a small part becomes a part of the whole. And a moment becomes part of the movement that God started when time first came to be.

Babies are a part of God's plan, and they are all unique and precious. They are the past, making it into the present, to get ready for the future. God has a marvelous way of interconnecting moments!

My father was in the service of the U.S. Navy, and he was stationed in Kodiak, Alaska. Kodiak is the largest island in the Aleutian chain.

It is a mountainous region, with abundant wildlife, sparsely dotted with human inhabitants—with the exception of the naval base. It is a place where God used nature's paintbrush to full advantage, with steep mountains peeking out from the stormy seas. The wind that blows there brings the smells of mountain air fragrant with pine and fir trees mixed with the salty sea air, and it teaches you God is in the wild places. Here, you can physically see, smell, and feel that God is God, and He is an awesome God.

It is here that my father had the opportunity to go to school and learn new skills. He was put on shore duty for an extended period. He wrote to my mother, who was in Iowa, and asked whether she would like to come to Alaska to visit for a month while he was on shore duty. My mother made plans to go visit my father, with the family doctor's approval. She took the train to the west coast and then boarded a ship from Seattle to head for Alaska.

From the ship, she thought it was odd that the houses were all one story. Until she found out the snow on the ground had buried the first floor, and what she was looking at was the second story of the houses. It was a lesson on Alaska in the early fall.

My father lived in off-base housing on the mountain overlooking the naval base. The road leading up the mountain was narrow and winding. One side was cut into the rocky face of the earth, and the other side overlooked deep ravines and rocky slopes, which show the heights you are leaving behind as you wind your way into the mountains. Halfway up, they built the small houses in an open meadow, which brought plenty of wildlife to peer into windows. Sometimes you had to wonder whether you were watching them, or they were watching you.

The Navy is watchful for their own and advised the sailors with wives in the off-base housing that this was still wilderness. They encouraged the wives to learn new skills for the area where they were living.

My mother, who was 5'2" tall and pregnant, did not pose a threat at first glance. My father taught her how to shoot a sawed-off shotgun, so she would feel safe. The first time she shot it, she got knocked off her feet and landed on her bottom. So, she had to compensate by using the fork of a tree until she got used to the weight and kick of the gun. My father taught her how to safely handle and clean the shotgun. As is required on base, you must announce that, "I have a gun. Halt or I'll shoot," three times before you fire your weapon. She was taught that if you aim it, be prepared to shoot it. They kept the gun filled with rock salt to keep the birds away from nesting under the eaves of the house.

My mother knew God would keep her safe, even in the wilderness. She told my father, "God doesn't send anything your way that you can't handle," and that he didn't need to worry.

My mother was just eight months pregnant when she experienced how God moves in mysterious ways. My father was away at work on the naval base, and my mother was cleaning the house. She would wash the dishes, floors, walls, and take all the throw rugs out and beat them over the clothesline. To her, it was as natural as breathing and a chore that would not even give one a passing sense that anything could go wrong.

But my mother was unaware of a man in the Navy who had not acclimated to military life and living in the wilderness. The Navy would later say he went off the deep end. He tore his clothes off and went screaming and running toward the off-base houses. He tried several doors, but the women had either seen or heard him and barricaded themselves into their homes.

My mother heard him, but because of the rugs couldn't see which direction he was coming from. She knew she wasn't going to stick around to find out what he was mad about and ran for the back door. When my mother started running, the movement caught the man's attention, and he started screaming incoherently and tried to overtake her.

My mother beat him to the door, slammed it, and barely got it locked before he hit the door at full speed. She was fumbling with the chain while he kept trying to knock the door down. He was tearing at the frame of the door. My mother yelled for him to leave and ran for the shotgun behind the kitchen door. The man had broken the door down by the time she reached the gun.

My mother said, "Halt or I'll shoot!" three times, with no break in between. He didn't halt, so she shot him with rock salt in the gun. The naked man screamed, turned toward the kitchen drawers, and pulled out a butcher knife. Before he could turn around, my mother shot him from behind. He fell to the floor, and my mother kicked the knife away from him. She placed the hot, hard steel of the gun on his back and said, "Halt means don't move!"

News of a madman in the off-base housing traveled fast as the other Navy wives called the base. My mother knew others had heard the man and the gunshots that followed. Navy wives are a family and look out for one another. Just as those who serve our country are family to each other, no one is left behind. My mother held the man there as women came running, looking through the open doorway and the door lying broken on the floor. She let them know she had him disarmed, and she needed someone to bring her a flat sheet to cover him up. They all asked her if she was okay. She said she was fine, but her stomach was upset. The other ladies had the presence of mind to know that my mother was probably going into labor, so they called my father to let him know to come home.

The military police were called and told to bring an ambulance, as there was a man down who had attempted to hurt several women. My father beat the ambulance up the narrow, winding road. He ran through the open back doorway to find my mother sitting on a kitchen chair she had pulled over, with the gun still aimed at the man lying out on the floor with a sheet over him. She told my father she was tired of standing, and she thought she needed to go and get checked at the hospital because her stomach was upset.

They called the naval hospital and told them that they were on the way to see whether they could stop her from going into labor. Both my parents knew that at eight months, it was too early for the baby to be born. By doctor's reasoning, she could just be having

Braxton Hicks contractions or false labor. This was my mother's first pregnancy, and most women having their first child don't know for sure when they are going into labor. Since it was her first pregnancy, they expected it to be slow, and they would have time to stop the labor.

By this time, the military police and the ambulance had arrived and had determined that the man's wounds were not life threatening. They asked about the weapon, but my mother told them she'd emptied it and had not reloaded the gun. She told them the man was down already, and she did not see a need to shoot the man when he was down. They were astonished that she'd kept a man down with an empty gun. But my mother told them, he didn't know that, and he was hurting badly enough he wasn't going to fight anymore.

They loaded the man on his side into the ambulance, and my mother and father followed it down the mountain to the hospital in their car. They got to the hospital and put my mother in a wheelchair, then started wheeling her to the maternity ward. My mother kept telling them the baby was coming, but they tried to reassure her that the doctor was going in to wash up, and he would be with her shortly to examine her. When they wouldn't listen, she stopped the wheelchair and told them to get the doctor—now. She saw the doctor coming down the hallway, his dripping hands bent up at the elbows. He called for some gloves. My mother told him she needed to push, and he realized the baby was crowning.

My mother said that she had more hands on her than she thought could go on a human body. She had people lifting, undressing, and propping her up all at the same time. She said it all happened so fast that the doctor bent down to catch me just as I was coming into this world. Then my mother did something unheard of—she grabbed me from the doctor to see whether I had all my fingers and toes.

Mother said the normal procedure during this time was the mother was put to sleep, and when she woke up, she would see her baby for the first time. My mother had the rare privilege of looking into the face of her newborn and touching me, even before I drew my first breath. The doctors and nurses were stunned but quickly told my mother she needed to hand the baby to the nurse, as she was sterile.

They measured me, weighed me, cleaned me up, and wrapped me in a blanket. They put me beside my mother, but my mother said she knew by how everyone was reacting in the room that something was not right.

My father was in the waiting room anxious for some news about what was happening. A nurse came in and called him to come with her; the doctor wanted to speak to him and my mother.

The doctor let them know that they had a daughter, and my mother was doing fine. But their baby was premature, very small, and was not going to live for very long. There was silence in the room, since no one knew what to say. Finally, in choked voices, they started asking questions about what my chances were.

My mother and father were still stunned by the news and reeling from what had transpired in the last twenty-four hours. The doctor pulled my father to the side and told him he needed to speak to him in private. He explained to my father that there was the indelicate matter of a burial to plan, and he didn't want to discuss it in front of my mother.

He asked whether my father had a chest of drawers. My father told him, "Yes, we have one for the baby, it's white." The doctor told him to take the top drawer, as it would be the smallest, and bring it to the hospital. Of course, my father was confused by this request. The doctor explained that I was too little for any coffin they had on the island. If my father brought the drawer, they would fill it with receiving blankets and get the bottom of a crate from the kitchen to nail to the drawer for the top of the coffin.

By this time, my father was just running on autopilot. He told the doctor, "I have to let my wife know where I am going, so she won't worry."

My father came into my mother's room, kissed her on the forehead, and told her he would be back, he had to go to the house.

My mother knew my father was very distraught over the news that this tiny baby of theirs had no chance to survive. But my mother knew he hadn't connected with this bundle of joy and told him he needed to hold me. So, she handed him the baby all wrapped up in a blanket, with only my little face showing.

My dad could not get over how small I was, and my mom told him, "But she has all her fingers and toes, and even though she is no bigger than a button, she has the cutest little face."

My father said, "That's because they wrapped her up so tight in the blanket, that's all you can see." My mother told him to keep me wrapped up so I wouldn't cry.

My father asked whether I had made any noise, and my mother told him that when they'd spanked me on my bottom, I'd made a loud noise.

My mother and father sat together in the hospital bed with their foreheads tenderly touching, looking at their new addition to the family. I managed to get a little hand out of the blankets and took ahold of my daddy's thumb. He marveled at how little it was and also the strength of my tiny grip. He told my mother how surprising this was to him. She said it shouldn't be surprising. I was the product of both of them, and they came from a long line of fighters. She wasn't about to give up on me, and she didn't want him to either.

"She was born alive, and any child of mine that was born alive is going to stay alive, so I can raise it right. And they are going to know, they are loved. My first born will not be the first baby that I lose. I am not willing to have that memory," my mother proclaimed.

The hospital staff went quietly past the room, not disturbing the occupants and giving them time to absorb the impending tragedy. Everyone knew what the outcome was going to be, and there was no other way that it could turn out. After all, the couple had clearly been told the baby was just eight months. The baby was fifteen inches long and weighed four pounds and six ounces. Hospital procedure required that as soon as I lost one ounce, I was to be put into an incubator. And every baby that the hospital had put into an incubator had died. Since all babies lose weight after they are born, it was inevitable what the outcome was going to be for this tiny, new life.

My mother knew my father was going back to the house, but she didn't know what the doctor had talked to him about. So, my mother wanted to keep my father's mind occupied on positive things. She made a list of things she wanted him to get while he was there. She let him know since there was a wood shortage on the island, because of the time of year, to just go ahead and nail the back door up and they would only have a front door for a while. She told him what types of clothing she wanted, and she said he would have to go to the store and buy doll clothes for the baby, because newborn sizes would be too big.

She told him not to worry, she was going to pray and everything would turn out all right. She asked him to take it easy going up the mountain, and when he came back down, she would have had time to have gotten a nap, as she was very tired. She said she knew why they call it labor—it is a lot of hard work, and when you get done, the baby and the momma need to get some rest.

She tried to put me in the crib that was in the room, but I was too small. So, she put me in a bassinet, which was also too big, but she put in a lot of rolled up blankets and diapers and put me in the center. I was going to have none of this; I started to cry, and so my dad knew I had a good set of lungs, to get this much noise out. My mom picked me up and realized I was hungry, and my dad told her, "Well, we know it's ours because we like to talk and eat, and she's letting us know she can do both, too."

My father kissed his girls goodbye and said he would be back after a bit. He left the hospital with a little bit of despair and a little more hope for the near future.

The nurses, seeing my father leave, came in to see how my mother was doing and found her feeding me. They asked her whether she would like something to eat. My mother told them that would be lovely, and when they came back with the food, they tried to take me away to the nursery. But my mother told them she wanted me to stay with her. The nurses allowed it, as they felt it would be better for the mother; so while my mother ate, I was falling asleep beside her in the bassinet.

My mother finished all the food and put the tray outside of the room. She got into bed and the next shift of nurses came in and checked on her. They glanced over at the crib, and no baby was in sight. They passed by the bassinet because it looked like it just had blankets and diapers inside. They told my mother to get some sleep, and they would wake her up when my father returned. They shut the curtains, so it would be easier for her to sleep, and shut the door.

My mother drifted off to sleep, listening to the short, whistling baby breaths coming from the bassinet beside her bed. She was awakened by a light brighter than day—the light filling her room. She saw three figures appear out of this light, and she knew she was in the presence of angels. She knew before they spoke that they were there to take the child home. She went to her knees in front of the bassinet and begged for them not to take the child. She told them that she and my father had big plans for a large family of twelve children, and this was her first born. She wouldn't be able to handle them taking me away. That I was loved, and she would take good care of me, and then she stopped in mid-sentence. She stood up, put her hand on the bassinet, and told the angels this: "You are not interested in the plans of man, but you are in what God wants." One of the angels told her God wanted me to come home and not suffer the pain of going into the incubator and slowly dying.

My mother told the angels to go back to God and tell Him that if He allowed this child to live, she would raise it for Him, and she would grow up knowing what God had done. The angels left for a short time and then came back. They told my mother God had accepted her covenant with Him. She was to understand that she was giving something up to receive the blessing.

Everybody who follows God gets a choice at least once—to stay or go to heaven. My mother gave up her choice to save me, so when

God called her home, she had to go. She requested that she be able to say goodbye to her family and friends before she died, and God granted her wish. The angels let my mother know because I had been saved to follow God, angels would watch over me and keep me from harm. My mother was to understand that there were going to be hardships, but I would persevere. Then the angels left her, and she was filled with such wonderful peace and love that she drifted off to sleep.

My father had gotten up the mountain and found some of his neighbors trying to shoo some birds out of his house. They got the birds out with brooms and dishcloths waving wildly about their heads. With some help, my dad got the back door nailed up and secured. He procured the articles my mother had requested and asked some of the neighbor ladies where he could get some doll clothes. He took the top drawer out of the baby chest and loaded the car up with his list of needed materials.

As he was loading everything into the car, he suddenly got a sense that everything was going to be all right. He felt as if a heavy burden had suddenly been taken away. So, he headed back down the mountain with a lighter spirit than when he had traveled up.

By the time he got back to the hospital with everything, he was feeling a little tired. Not wanting to disturb my mother, he asked a nurse how my mother and I were doing. They said he could go in, as my mother had just woken up from her nap.

He peeked into the room, and my mother could hardly contain herself as she told him about her three heavenly visitors. My father didn't quite know what to make of this, but my mother asked him, didn't he feel better about their baby's chances? He said he did. That was my mother's proof to him that what she was saying was real.

The little top drawer that was to be my coffin became my bed. God sent a different perspective, when you call on Him for help and guidance, and that makes all the difference in the world.

Psalm 84:11
For the Lord God is a sun and shield; the Lord bestows favor and honor; no good thing does he withhold from those whose walk is blameless.

Psalm 103:2-3
Praise the Lord, O my soul, and forget not all his benefits— who forgives all your sins and heals all your diseases.

Chapter Two

God Watches Over Me

My parents stayed in Alaska for a year, and instances in my early life caused people to marvel at me. Many Navy men brought their families and babies together in groups. My parent's friends brought their babies when they hung out. I was the smallest and baldest baby. When I was born, I had black, curly hair, but it all fell out. My mother, not to be outdone by the little problem of no hair, would still stick pink bows wherever she could get them to stay. I was constantly wearing lacy dresses with bows, ribbons, and braided edgings. People would still come up to her and say that I was a cute boy, and it used to get her so mad. After all, what baby boy wears pink?

Such a new, small family, and we were all facing obstacles. People were amazed by my mother's ability to be happy and positive when friends close to her knew what she and my father were facing together.

I became allergic to the new wonder drug, sulfa, and had been very sick afterwards. Doctors were always telling my parents it's a miracle I was still alive.

My mother had gone to the doctor and was told that she couldn't have any children. She had a tipped uterus and scar tissue from when she had scarlet fever as a child. Mother told the doctor that she'd had a baby anyway, and the doctor said she wouldn't be able to carry another baby full term, and I would be their last child. My father told my mother that half the fun was in the trying.

In addition to my frailties and my mother's diagnosis, my father started having troubles with his health. He went to the naval doctor, and they gave him some disheartening news. His health had been going downhill for some time, but he had kept working and taking care of his family. One of his kidneys was failing. It was working at thirty percent, and the other was slowly deteriorating. He was told that he didn't have long to live—after all, nobody could live without functioning kidneys. They explained my father would slowly get worse until they put him in the hospital, where all they would be able to do was keep him comfortable. They told my mother to go home and love him while she could because she wouldn't have him for very long.

Mother told the doctors that God answers prayers, and she and God were going to keep my father alive until the doctors and technology could figure out a way to help him. The doctors told her it would be way off in the future, if it was ever possible. My mother told them anything is possible with God.

With this news, my father was told he couldn't stay in the Navy. The military goes through a medical discharge process that is not fast, but it's done precisely and in triplicate. Shore duty for a sailor is a letdown when the sea can no longer be your home. God sends you a detour sometimes, and you have to remember to be ready to adjust to what God has planned. Instead of complaining and worrying about why and standing in the middle of the road, learn to steer a new course when a curve comes in your path. It takes a whole lot less time to change direction than to stop and turn around, fighting against the right of way. God's way is always the best way to go. Just follow Him, and you won't worry anymore about right ways.

My parents let their families know back in Iowa about the things that were going on in the wilderness of Alaska. My parents told them they were going to take each day as it came and pray and let God take care of the rest. They didn't keep it a secret, but they didn't dwell on their troubles. They let God be God and knew He would take care of them.

Our home was small, but it was filled with love. In this environment, I was someone with high energy and determination. And limitations didn't stop my need to explore and expand my knowledge of my world. Where I didn't grow in height, I did put on weight. With the other children around, I wanted to be able to do what they were doing. So, I stood at nine months and was able to run at ten-and-a-half months. My father used to say, "Merrily has two speeds—full speed and stop." I didn't really walk; I ran, and I was so small I would be able to go under coffee tables and kitchen tables until I was two-and-a-half years old.

I was curious and into everything, which kept my parents on their toes, for I could get lost easily with my being so small. But small didn't stop me from doing things. I just learned to do them differently. For instance, I would crawl up or down stairs, because my legs weren't long enough to step up or down to the next step. I learned from the start to problem solve and do it quickly. I could sit for hours in a patch of sunlight, playing with a stuffed bear, and fall asleep on top of him, catch a cat nap, and wake back up and play in the same spot. If there was some excitement going on, I had to be in the thick of things, so I didn't miss anything.

My mother put bells on my shoes so she could find me, but she told my father it drove her crazy when I was running around, but then she'd panic when she didn't hear them ringing. My dad told her I had music wherever I went, and my mom told him, "It's more like noise when you are in the house by yourself with her." But it gave her an idea. I loved music, so she turned on the radio, and I stayed close by as long as the music played. The musical bells on my shoes were taken off.

I gave my parents many challenges as I grew. I had the uncanny knack for being able to absolutely intrigue and be a pied piper to everything that ran, crept, crawled, or flew. I wanted to be around them, and they wanted to be with me. God has a way of getting you prepared for things to come.

In Alaska, there are the Eskimo sled dogs—the Husky and the Malamute. Across the street from our house was a family that had taken in a Husky for a pet. He would sit out in the snow very content and watch the goings on in the neighborhood. While he was watching the neighbors, I was watching him through the living room window. Now, my mother was a very protective mother, and she tried her best to keep me from harm or hurt. No matter the method or how strong the desire is to accomplish this feat, failure is just around the corner. You can't hold back the tide with a broom, and you can't stop a child from being curious.

My mother had just come from the grocery store and had one hand around the brown paper sack and one hand bent down holding my hand. This was an uncomfortable stretch for my mother to hang on to each equally well. I was flexible and fast, and she was not prepared for the speed that was pent up in me from being still in the car for so long. I saw the dog across the street lying in the snow, and I got it in my head to go play—now.

I had on a one-piece light pink snowsuit with white boots. Now this is quite fetching fashion wise, but it doesn't do a thing for visibility in high snows. A snowplow was coming down the street—the type in large snowfall areas where full grown men have to use the ladders on the side to get into the cab. I was past my mother's reach through the snow. I was walking on top of a thin, hard crust, and I stayed on top because of my light weight. My mother was waving and screaming at the snowplow operator to stop, but he couldn't hear her. And her weight was just dragging her deeper into the snow.

The dog across the street saw what was happening and knew I was in danger. He flattened out in a full run and came across the street, grabbed my snowsuit-covered arm, and pulled me away from the street. I was looking up from the snow-covered ground at a furry face licking me and then my frightened mother pulling me up in her arms.

My mother told the dog to follow her, and he did, very happy that she was pleased with him knocking down the wayward child. My father missed a steak dinner that night, but one dog was very full and satisfied at a job well done. After this, my mother saved all the bones for him, and he was a very well-praised dog for his heroism.

This was only the beginning of a lifelong cooperation between me and animals—a connection that God created. Animals have saved my life many times over the years, and I have saved some of their lives. My ability to relate with them has continued to amaze people. Not just domestic animals but the wild things, too.

I remember going to the zoo in Seattle, Washington with my mother. She put me in a stroller to contain me and keep watch over me. When you strap a child in, you expect the child will remain strapped in until you take the child out. That sense of security is a reliable assumption when dealing with children and child safety products.

My mother quite happily strapped me in, put the baby bag under the stroller, and started pushing it toward the large cat exhibit. My mother recognized how much I loved animals and thought this would be something I would long remember. She was right, but not quite the way she thought. I had a more adventurous twist to put on our expedition to the zoo.

The animals were in large cages with black iron bars. There were some low-lying shrubs around the base of these outdoor exhibits and then a roped off section that was at the edge of the sidewalk, allowing for observation without danger to people or animals. Large signs posted everywhere said not to feed the animals, and of course the plaques that told what animals were inside and some facts about them. My mother, who was interested in expanding my knowledge, was reading the plaque to me about the occupant in each cage, and this is where they live in the wild. I was pointing and laughing and just absolutely thrilled to be so close to something I loved. When my mother thought she had sufficiently watched a cage long enough, she would move onto the next one and repeat the process.

We had seen the lions, leopards, and the tigers. Now my mother used to say that I had the uncanny ability to know when I was being watched. So obviously it also meant I knew when I wasn't being watched. My mother's perspective was I did it when she wasn't looking. I did it simply because I wasn't done looking, and I wanted a closer look.

I wanted to see more of the tiger lying up next to the cage. He had positioned himself in the shade next to the water, with his body pressed against the bars. His long, striped tail, as thick as a broom handle, was outside the bars slowly moving back and forth. It was an open invitation to a child of high interest and unending curiosity.

My mother was moving on to the next exhibit and not really paying attention to a child calling for a big kitty. She thought I was looking at the one we were going to, not the one we had already seen. My mother had to make a turn in toward the next exhibit, and pushing a stroller, she had to lift the front and turn with the back wheels. When this process is being done, the weight in the stroller is shifted and feels lighter, and I chose that moment to simply slip out of the strap and walk over to the tiger cage.

My mother's view was obstructed by the stroller, and she never felt the change in weight. By the time she made the turn, she didn't feel the need to look back. So, she didn't see her daughter walk under the rope barrier, over to the tiger's tail, and start scratching it. The tiger heard all this giggling and felt something pleasantly scratching where he couldn't reach. A loud rumbling sound started to come out from deep within, and he closed his eyes and clenched and unclenched his big claws, as he relished this delightful child who had found just the right spot.

My mother was at the next exhibit along the path and slightly higher from the last exhibit. She said she looked down in the stroller, and to her utter shock, I was not there. The straps were still in place, but I was not in the stroller. She started looking underneath and calling my name. I, being a dutiful child, answered with, "Hi, Mommy," but not in a place where my mother wanted me to be. She always said she knows angels watch over children, and I had to be someone who God blessed because I was put in some places where angels fear to tread. She doesn't remember going downhill, but she remembers reaching underneath the roped barrier to grab a piece of my clothing and trying to get me closer, so she could get me away from the tiger. I remember being pulled, and then I'm in my mother's arms, and there is the sound of a tiger roaring. It might be that he wanted a tail scratcher for a little longer, but my mother always contended he wanted a little snack before supper.

When fear subsides and distance is between you and what you fear, you can get a different perspective. My mother would tell that story to let people know I had a connection with animals, and there was no fear in regards to animals. I was often asked growing up why, since they were bigger, stronger, faster, and able to cause harm to me. I would tell them that somehow, we know we mean each other no harm, and we each have mutual respect for one another.

Psalm 121:7-8
The Lord will keep you from harm—he will watch over your life; the Lord will watch over your coming and going both now and forevermore.

Proverbs 18:10
The name of the Lord is a strong tower; the righteous run to it and are safe.

Chapter Three

The Merry-Go-Round of Life

Have you ever been on a merry-go-round? It goes around and around, and portions go up and down, all while music is playing. It's my favorite ride because it reminds me of life on Earth. The world keeps spinning no matter if you are having ups and downs or staying level. This might give you a different perspective when going through life.

The Holy Spirit is like the music; it surrounds you, and all you have to do to be comforted is to listen. Sometimes life will hand you a plate full of unpleasantness, and you have to make decisions you are not prepared to make. When that time comes, stop, take a breath, and review the pros and cons or assets and liabilities. This is a way to take the turmoil out of decisions, and you can find great peace in knowing you made an informed choice.

I ask God to help me see what He wants me to do. Sometimes, God doesn't want you to take the easy way. Remember, the only way to get an easy way is somebody has to do it hard first. Then tell everybody. Some will do it the same way because you did it that way. The mighty oak comes from a little acorn, and the only way it grows is because of its struggle to break through the ground. Still others will try to improve the task and make it better and easier.

I have seen the storm clouds surround me, and it becomes darker and duller, like a faded newspaper; and then sometimes the sun peeks through, and the contrast is so dramatic that your eyesight seems like it has gotten better instantly. You feel more alive and real in that moment than the moment before because you are witnessing God's power. You have trouble or danger encompassing you; but God is above it and beyond it, and sometimes He gives you the privilege to see for yourself. You have to have faith that the acorn, when it falls to the ground, will grow—as it is covered by the soil, and you can't see. When it pushes up out of the ground, then the seeing becomes knowing. God is like that. At first, we have to have faith He is there; and when we experience God, then we know He is there.

In our own human way, we try to make things easier. If something does not work like we expect, our mind goes to simple solutions. It is also to our favor if it is not hard or difficult. We can quickly go back to our regular routine. We are not puppets or robots that are controlled. We are not mice in a maze looking for a small piece of cheese. We can be still and make a different outcome by using the steppingstones across the stream of life's whirling eddies.

When an obstacle gets in my way, I can go around, go over, go under, go through, or I can remove it. It does not make it a stop sign. Even when you stop, you wait and then make a decision of how to move on. It is simply part of the learning process we have in life.

Growing up, I soon became aware that I was getting sick more often than siblings or children at school. I got ear infections and sore throats easily, and it kept me from school and fun activities. I got dizzy spells, and it was just thought to be a side effect of the ear infections. I started having fainting spells, and it was assumed it was over exertion or the weather. My not being able to sit or stand straight was annoying, since I leaned all the time. In all my pictures, I was leaning to the side. It was thought to be an after effect of my many ear infections, which put me at a permanent tilt. My being born too early had doctors convinced it was the reason for my allergies and easily getting sick.

My parents would ask the doctors why I was sick and what could be done to prevent another episode. The ear infections were most likely caused by windy conditions, they were told. I was promptly wearing hats and scarfs when there was an outdoor adventure. In the summer, I had to wear a hat to keep me cool. Too hot or too cold aggravated my symptoms, and eliminating or checking the severity to a tolerable level was the plan. The doctors were treating the symptoms as a way to get me on the road to recovery. If I got sick from the medicine I was given, it was added to the list of allergies.

I was an active child, and I worked with all of my restrictions. The doctors were sure I would outgrow some of my health issues. After a while, it was clear I would need to take precautions to prevent symptoms that did not go away. I was a puzzle to doctors, with multiple symptoms that didn't add up. They were looking for that one missing piece, which would bring the full picture together.

I inadvertently gave them the clue while I was telling the doctor what happened. I said at the end, "…just like my grandpa and dad." The doctor had been nodding his head and writing down notes. He looked up and said for me to sit up on the examining table. He listened to my chest with his stethoscope until he found the right spot. I got a turn to listen to my heart as well. I asked why I'd heard an extra sound. The doctor said I had a heart valve that wasn't closing all the way. It was what my grandfather and father had, and it was called a left mitral valve prolapse.

I asked whether it would go away on its own. The doctor explained it was highly likely to be hereditary, and it was progressive. There were steps to prolong life with a pig's valve replacement, artificial valve, and then a pacemaker. This is what eventually would be the pathway my grandfather and father had to take for the same ailment. My mother was discouraged at the news, but I was happy. I had a name for what was causing me problems. I had a clear path of what it was, what was restricted, and most important what I could do. In the Bible, it says if you can name it, you can claim victory over it in Jesus's name. It did keep progressing as predicted, but not to the extent of my grandfather and father. I didn't require any surgery to fix the defective valve in my heart. Miracles were continuing to be a part of my life.

As I got older, my different health issues would put me in the hospital. I knew God was watching over me, and He would find a way where human beings were getting frustrated and perplexed. I asked God to help the doctors find out what was wrong with me. I had been to so many doctors and found out what I didn't have but not what I had. Elimination of the possibilities is a way to get to the right answer, but it takes a long time and lots of tests to go through.

The doctors went on a quest to find out what was wrong with me. My family doctor sent me to Iowa City to a hospital there. They found out my eyes were getting worse because my retinas were stretched as far as they could go, and both my eyes had small tears in the bottom. They gave me the grim news that my retinas could become detached, and I would not be able to see. There was a fifty/fifty chance a surgery could help. I was told not to get hit in the head or be in any kind of accident, to give me a better chance at having vision for a while longer.

After the results of the tests came back, my family doctor said he wanted me to go to the Mayo Clinic in Rochester, Minnesota for a week. My grandmother agreed to go with me, and my mom watched my son, Clifford, for me. We checked into the hospital, and they gave me the itinerary of what they planned for each day and what kind of doctor would be seeing me. We stayed at a hotel, and I came to the hospital every day to be poked, prodded, and examined. At the end of the week, they sat me down and let me know the results.

I had vertigo since birth; my allergy to sulfa had affected my kidneys; and I had sponge kidneys, which stored the sulfa and attached itself to protein. So, when my kidneys could hold it no more, they would flush out the sulfa, and I lost protein at the same time and in large quantities. My allergy was now to sulfa, sulfite, sulfate, and sulfur.

I asked what I could do about what they had found. Sulfur is in the air, soil, and water. It is a preservative and an additive in multiple things like medicine and food. There was no way to get around it; I would continue to have this problem. I would have an option to drink water that was purified by reverse osmosis and charcoal filtered, and this would relieve a lot of the problem.

I sat there in the doctor's office as they explained everything. There was a numbness that enveloped me, as I tried to comprehend what all this meant. When the doctor paused and asked whether I had any questions about their findings, I asked what they had found out with the psychological testing I had taken. He said it was no surprise I was an introvert but did extrovert things. He asked why I was curious about those particular findings. I told him that I wanted to thank him, and I shook his hand. The doctor was startled and asked me to explain.

I said, "You have put a name to things that have affected me, some since birth. It can no longer be said—oh, she just gets dizzy or she faints a lot or it is all in her head." The doctor asked why this would make a difference. I said, "I have listened to people all my life as they have dismissed me for getting sick or hurt or thinking I had to be faking some illness. My nature is shy and quiet, and yet I do the opposite in the spectrum. You have proven God is in my life, and He takes care of me. I have some purpose God keeps me here for, and because you have given them names, I can claim victory over them. Satan is running from a beating." I told the doctor he had given me joy, and I was very grateful.

Surprised, he questioned whether I was glad I was sick. I said, "Knowing is freedom, and now I just work within the framework I have been given." The doctor asked why I did not just ask God to take away the illness. I said, "God gives these things to me to slow me down and to know that without God, I would not be here.

Where I am weak, God makes me strong; and where I am strong, God keeps me humble."

The doctor shook his head and told me this was the strangest consultation he had ever had. He asked whether I had any other concerns. I told him yes, I did have one. The doctor perked up right away and asked me to tell him my concern. I asked, "How do you explain to a child what is going on with the main caregiver in their life, without making them fearful or anxious?" The doctor asked the age of the child and a little about him. He said that stress had been a major factor I needed to get relief from, and he said the best way was to lay down the rules from the start.

I asked for suggestions, and he said, "Go home and tell your son this: Rule number one, Momma makes the rules. Rule number two, you follow the rules. Rule number three, don't forget rule number one and two." The doctor said to be honest and up front with Clifford about my health and what steps were being taken, and I should not have any trouble with Clifford getting upset. The doctor said I was the one Clifford was looking to, to see whether it bothered me or affected me in an adverse way. He told me that my attitude would make the difference, and he was very happy to have met me.

I had confirmed why he had become a doctor, and he was glad he could still make a difference that was positive. He let me know all their findings would be sent to my family doctor, and I should set up an appointment with my doctor when I got back home.

I thanked him again, and I walked out of his office with a lighter step and spirit.

When I got back home, I took his advice and told Clifford what the doctor said. Clifford took it all in stride and asked, "Does this mean you aren't going to die?"

I said, "It means that I am not dead yet."

Clifford asked, "How long will you live?"

I said, "Just as long as God needs me here, I can stay. When God is done, He will call me home to heaven."

Clifford thought for a minute and said, "Well, you have to stay and take care of me until I get big, so you will be here for a while."

That satisfied my son, and he agreed the rules were simple and he could remember them, too.

My family doctor was very interested in the results and decided to put me on some medicine for my heart. Tenormin would slow my heart rate down, and twenty minutes after taking it, I was asleep—the kind of deep sleep that is very difficult to wake from, and so I adjusted the time I took it. I could wake up early the next morning, with no trouble. I was determined to work within the timeframe that best suited my medicine and keep my family comfortable with the adjustments that had to be made to keep me healthy.

I was raised to do your very best, to try—because success or failure begins with trying. You see, the turtle never gets anywhere unless he sticks his neck out. My parents told all their children to be the very best they could be, and that is all anyone can ask of you. They said they didn't care whether you were a ditch digger—be the very best one you could be, and they would be proud of us. It is not your station in life that makes you great. It has always been what is inside of you that counts, and what you share with this world.

Romans 8:28
And we know that in all things God works for the good of those who love him, who have been called according to his purpose.

Ephesians 2:8-9
For it is by grace you have been saved, through faith—and this not from yourselves, it is a gift of God—not by works, so that no one can boast.

Chapter Four

God Is Greater than Cancer

I had just begun writing a book about my life when I found out that sometimes you must step back before you can go forward. I found a profound lesson on life. If God calls you to do something, will you do it no matter what?

I had many times found lumps. I went to the doctor, and they did needle aspirations on them. It was uncomfortable but no big deal. I went to the doctor to have one done. I explained that ever since I'd fallen and hit the banister one time, the muscles healed but there was still a hard lump. The doctor examined it and said she wanted x-rays. It was bigger than one they had done needle aspirations on, and possibly I would need to have it removed. She thought she would send me to get a biopsy of the tissue, just for safe measure.

I went where they told me to go. They did a mammogram first, and then I went and got a biopsy. It was done under local anesthesia and in an office. They found another lump behind the first one and said they had not seen it with x-rays or the mammogram. They said while they were already there, they would go ahead and do this one also. When they were through, they told me when they got the results, they would call my doctor. My doctor would then give me the results.

I went on with my normal routine. I was in the parking lot of a business while someone I was helping was inside for a job interview. I got a call from the doctor's office, and they asked whether I wanted to come in or if I wanted them to tell me the results over the phone. I said they could tell me the results over the phone. Then they asked whether I was alone or if I had someone with me. I told them I was by myself but was waiting for somebody to finish an appointment. They told me the results came back, and it was cancer. There was a pause, and they asked whether I was okay. I said I was, and I asked what the next step was. They needed me to come in, and they were going to start getting appointments set up. They asked when I could come in. I let them know that I was helping someone right now, but I would finish and then come in.

They apologized that it was not good news. I said, "It is good news. From the perspective that we found it, and we just need to go from here." They said I was taking it especially well. I let them know, "I am right now, and that is the main thing, and then focus on the next step."

I got off the phone and sat in the car. I decided I would wait until I could see the doctor and go from that point. I had people relying on me that I needed to finish helping. I did not say anything when they got back into the car. I felt as though I did not have all the information yet, and it would be very upsetting news. I took them back to their house and went to the doctor's office.

The doctor's office was frantically trying to set up appointments with other specialists. They explained this needed to be done quickly. When I was given all the information, I asked whether I should tell people. They said they felt it was a good idea, as I would need a lot of support. This was going to affect my life, and people in it needed to know.

I went about telling people, and I spent a lot of time consoling distraught people who could not believe it was happening to me.

Some took it harder than others. I told them I had to go to the doctor and specialists, and they would let me know what my options were.

I wanted to wait until I had all the information before I told my kids. I went to the surgeon, and he said there were two options. I could go with a lumpectomy, just taking out the lumps, or a mastectomy, removing the breast and lymph glands. On most people, he said it was 50/50. In my case, he had more concerns. One lump was very close to my chest wall, and there was the possibility that it had spread to other parts of the body. He was leaning toward the mastectomy, but it was still my choice.

I was asked if I had a husband. I told him, "No, I am divorced." I was asked if I had a fiancé. I said, "No."

Then I was told I would have to make the decision myself, as it seems like any other person would doubt their decision. I asked how long I had to make a decision, and they gave me ten minutes. There was an urgency to get into surgery, and available appointments were filling up. So, I was left alone for ten minutes to decide which plan I wanted to follow.

I reminded myself that I was not alone, and that God is wiser than me. I prayed and asked God to show me the way. I recalled all the times I had gotten hit on the right side, and how the right side was smaller because of the poison from a bee sting. I said, "God, all along you have shown me how to live with it being less than the other side. All the needle aspirations were on the right side. I read in your Word it says that if a part of your body sins, to cut it off. It is better to go to heaven missing that part than to continue to sin." I said, "Thank you for helping me to know what you want me to do."

The doctor came back in, and I said, "I choose the mastectomy."

The first opening for surgery was before Christmas, and I said, "I cannot do that to my children." The next opening was just before New Year's. I told them I would do that one.

I gathered my family and friends together and explained to them that I wanted a combined front when I told my children. I had let the children know I was having tests done and was waiting for the results. I went to the school and spoke with the principal, counselors, and teachers. And everyone agreed to meet with the children together. When everybody was together, I told the children what the results were, the decision I'd made, and that I was going to have an operation. I said, "Everyone in this room is here to help you and answer what questions we can."

The kids had a few, but for the most part they were calm. The principal said he wished he had a recording of what I'd said. He said I'd showed great wisdom in how I'd told my children. I thanked him and explained that I had been open and honest with them on what was happening. I waited until I had all the information and support before I told them this part.

Joy, my daughter, asked whether I was scared. I said, "No, I am trusting God is taking care of me. I have found it is more the fear of others to ease that is more frequent. I know God is not done with me. He has a purpose I have to fulfill."

I let the church know I was going in for surgery and when. I told them that I knew God was with me, and I was already healed. I proclaimed that by Jesus wounds I am already healed in the name of Jesus. People prayed for me and asked to be kept informed of how I was doing. I told the pastor I had no fear of going into surgery. I knew everything would be okay.

Arrangements were made, and things were set up so that if I were incapacitated, things would continue on and keep a stable environment for the children. My ex-husband Peter was watching the children, as I would be in the hospital for two days. I had people lined up for care and bills all taken care of before going to the hospital. Many well-wishers were calling and making sure I was still in good spirits. Pastor went to the hospital to pray for me before the surgery. I told everyone it was going to be all right. I was at peace, and I was not afraid.

When the surgery was done, I woke up and people came into the recovery room to see me. Everyone was glad I was okay. The nurse came in and said that when the anesthesia wore off, I was to let them know my pain level. She asked on a scale of 0–10, with 10 being the most pain I'd ever felt, where was my pain level. I said zero, and she said to not be brave. They had things for pain that were prescribed to me if I needed it. I said, "Thank you, but I don't have any pain."

When I had recovered, they put me in another room. They told me to let them know if I needed to use the bathroom or if I started to hurt. It is important to walk and get your body to start functioning back to normal as soon as possible.

The surgeon came in and said everything went well, and the surgery was a success. He explained that the cancer doctor would come see me, and we would have some follow-up appointments. I could not drive for two weeks, so someone would have to get me to my appointments. I thanked him for taking such good care of me.

I had nurses keep checking on me, and one came in and asked to know my pain level. I said I was fine. The nurse insisted that if I had any discomfort, to tell her. I said, "Well, I have no pain, but I do have some discomfort." She was anxious to know where, so I started to point to it and then said, "Oh, never mind, it is just the string on my gown. I was lying on it." She tried to keep a straight face. She said, "Excuse me," and after she stepped out, I heard her laughing in the hall. She started to come back in twice and had to leave when she saw my face. The third time she got back in to finish checking my vitals. I said, "Laughter is good medicine for nurses, too." She agreed as she was leaving, and I heard her laughing in the hall again.

When people came to see me, I told them I had no pain. I said it was a gift from God. This was major surgery, and I told them God was healing me. People would nod their heads and say it was good to have a positive attitude. I told them a positive attitude is nothing without God.

At that point, I had not looked at my surgery site, and I thought I'd better because they were asking whether I had questions about it. I went into the bathroom and looked into the mirror. I started to cry, but then I pulled myself up and said, "No, this is what God said to do, and you made a choice to follow God. This is not a time for tears or sadness, but of joy that He saw fit to let me stay a little while longer. God sent me no pain as a sign that He is with me. I will just lean on Him to help me get through the tough times to come."

When I got home, I had exercises to do. I had been trained on the drain tubes and what to look for as danger signs—where and when I would have to return to the doctor. I called the people that had said they would be helping me with my care. The insurance kept turning me down, so I had no one with me. I was limited in what I could lift, and I sent everyone away because it had all been worked out with people the insurance would not cover.

A friend came out of a program he was in to help me. He stayed to help with cooking, cleaning, and the children. He said I helped everybody; it was time to get help back. He stayed until I could do things on my own.

I had a follow-up with the doctors, and they wanted to look at the surgery site and my range of motion. I started to take my coat off, and I put my hands behind my back. The surgeon asked whether we had done a mastectomy. I told him yes, and he said first, my arm had not atrophied, so he could not tell which side. Second, that I should not yet be able to put my arms behind my back. No pain was also a major triumph, which could not be explained.

I said, "God is a miracle-working God." The doctor said he agreed, and it showed up in my case. He told me eight out of eight free. I did not comprehend, and he clarified that eight lymph glands had been removed, and all eight were cancer free. All my tests were good, and he said the cancer doctor would see me next.

I had more tests run, and when I saw the cancer doctor, he had options for me. Chemotherapy, radiation, estrogen pills, or nothing was on my list. I listened to all my options and all the percentages if I did each one. I chose to do nothing more. He asked me why this was my choice. I said I had gone with the one that gave me peace. I told him that I'd come into the world with zero chance to live, so any of those options were better than that. I went to all my follow-ups and was diagnosed cancer free.

I told everyone God had made me cancer free. There was lots of praise for a God that saves our souls and heals our bodies. Nothing is too much for the God I serve. I went for check-ups and tests—all of them came back that everything was good.

Later, I found a lump between my ribs. I had it checked by my family doctor. My insurance company had dropped me, and the cancer doctor could not examine me until it was cleared and my insurance was restored. I was able to get the insurance issue cleared up. I went and had the cancer doctor look at the lump, and he said for me to go to the surgeon. The surgeon said we needed to remove it to be sure. I let people know, and I told them God was going to heal me. This lump was between my ribs but not attached, and it was cancer. It was explained that I'd dodged a bullet because it had not spread.

I was told by the cancer doctor that I was going to be on the estrogen pill because there was a 100% chance the cancer would be back if I did not. I told them God did not give me any pain, and I would be cancer free again.

I was allergic to the pill I took, but the cancer doctor gave me medicine for my symptoms. I told them if I am allergic, it will not do what it is supposed to do. I took it as they told me to and as prescribed. I was told it was better to fight symptoms than cancer. I went back for each appointment. They ran all kinds of tests. I was cancer free and pain free.

I was watchful and found something a third time. It was so small I had to put my finger on it so they could find it. Ultrasounds and a biopsy followed. Again, it was cancer. I went for surgery and because it was in the muscle tissue, it left a raised scar this time. I went back to find out the results of all the tests. The cancer doctor told me it was confirmed the lump was cancer in my chest and no more cancer was found there. He asked if I was feeling pain anywhere else. I said, "No, I have no pain anywhere."

He said that was strange since the cancer had moved to my bone, and it was in my hip and my spine. He told me cancer likes to move to bone, blood, lungs, heart, and brain. I said, "Then it is a good thing that I had cancer show up in my chest, so you could find where it moved to in my body."

I asked what was next, and he said, "You will no longer take the estrogen pill." He wanted me to do radiation and was looking at giving me some stronger cancer medicine. I would go to radiation for a consultation. They made the appointment as soon as possible. I went, and they explained what it was and what it did. There were all kinds of possible side effects, and I had to sign papers. I would be having a high pinpoint dose for ten days.

It did not take long, and I could go about with the rest of my day. I would need to have tattoos, which I was not sure of, and they told me they were medical tattoos—dots to help them center the machine. This would essentially make the cancer stop growing further in those areas.

I went back to the cancer doctor after the radiation treatments. Radiation did make me tired, but I worked with how I felt and still helped people. The cancer doctor wanted me to take two pills and said they would keep the cancer from coming back. I was leery of taking them, and so I had people try to talk me into it. My heart was not settled on what they were telling me. I was told to take the pills if I wanted to live longer. They were chemotherapy in a pill form. The side effects filled pages.

I prayed about what to do. I told God I did not want fear to make me decide. I wanted God to show me what was best for me and all my other health issues. I felt at peace when I decided not to take the pills.

The cancer doctor wanted me to take them and asked me why this was my choice. I said I believed God was directing me to not take this medicine. I wanted to lead a normal life. I was told normal went out the door the day I was diagnosed with cancer. I had stage four breast cancer that had metastasized. I said, "God is greater than cancer." My doctor said he had people who were Christians die from cancer. I said, "Hallelujah, my mother was one of them." He told me people come in there who run marathons. They are diagnosed with cancer, and a few years later they die.

I said, "God has a purpose for my life, and it is not done yet."

The doctor told me that there was a 90% chance this cancer would kill me off in five years. He was going to set up an appointment a year from now, and he thought I would get worse without medicine. He said I would be in pain, and he would put me in the hospital and then hospice. He felt I would not last the year. I said I would see him next year, and he said it would be a miracle if I did.

I said I felt I was already. I said, "Cancer is just a label of how I could die. It can be said I could walk out of here and be run over or have a heart attack. God is the one who orders my steps, and He is the only one who knows when I will die."

This same doctor knew from the beginning that I was diagnosed with breast cancer, stage four. I should have been in so much pain that I would be in a pain management regimen in the hospital, while visitors came to say goodbye to me. I had been cancer free twice and had no pain. I was told I was a miracle. I am still a miracle of God. In my chest, I am cancer free. I have cancer in my bone, in my hip, and in my spine. They did not remove it with surgery. It is there and not growing where they radiated it.

I listened to people who have done research on my behalf. I started a regimen of herbs and supplements, which help fight cancer. I walked more and stayed active, helping people whenever I could. I am not done until God says I'm done.

When the next year's appointment with the cancer doctor came around, the doctor thought I had taken his advice and taken the pills he prescribed. I said I had not taken them. He asked what I was doing, and I said I had added herbs and supplements to my diet. He asked about how I dealt with the pain, and I once again explained that I had no pain.

The doctor said the test results came back, and I had no new cancer. He informed me the insurance would no longer be able to take me unless I could pay out of pocket expenses. The doctor asked if I had any assets to sell or a house to mortgage. He said he could not see me again until I could pay for my treatments. I told him I had no way to pay, since I was low income. He said I could try my relatives and see if they could come up with the money needed. He would be happy to see me when money wasn't an issue. I thanked him for letting me know, and I walked out of his office. I could not make an appointment, so I gave the receptionist the paperwork and left.

People were asking me from church how well I had done this time. I let them know the cancer had not grown. The doctor was surprised I had not taken the medicine. But the doctor had a surprise of his own. Now I had to come up with the money myself for treatments because the insurance had informed him they would not cover me. Everyone wondered what I was going to do. I told them I know God has a plan. I have no way on my own to follow up on the demands the doctor has placed at my feet. God will show me what to do in His time. I was not going to stop helping people, and as long as my health would allow it, I was going to do my best to be a helper.

We are all dying, for we all return to the dust from which we came. But I can decide how my quality of life will be, and this is my choice. I want to continue to help others and to be a helper of those in need.

James 4:8
Come near to God and he will come near to you.

I Peter 2:24
He himself bore our sins in his body on the tree, so that we might die to sins and live for righteousness; by his wounds you have been healed.

Chapter Five

Why Not Treat All of Me?

When God looks at me, He sees all of me. He knows me inside out. He has my past, present, and future in His hands. I know God is above all things. He watches over my coming in and my going out. He cares about me. The all-knowing, all-seeing, and ever-present God loves me. What a mighty God I serve!

God is my helper. Since the health insurance could not be involved with my continuing condition of cancer, I gave it to God. Nothing humanly could be done, so I went on knowing God would make a way. God helped me with kidney stones. I was able to pass them on my own without a hospital stay. God helped me through a detached retina. I got the care I needed, and people showed up to help. God was there for both of my cataract surgeries and recovery. God did not let me down. He leads me through and back out on the other side. God provides and protects me because God is faithful.

With my eyes being able to see clearly again, I went back to helping people. Gradually, I felt it was becoming harder to stand or walk for any length of time. It reached a point where I needed to go see what was wrong. I went to my family doctor, and they felt I had overworked my muscles. I was told about some over the counter medicines to take to see if it helped. The more I moved, the worse I got. I went back to my doctor, and they felt it was a pinched nerve. They could give me a shot of pain medicine in my hip and pain pills to get back to my normal self. I went down the list of my allergies, and they said this would be a quick shot. I was to wait ten minutes, and then I could go home and rest for the remainder of the day.

I waited the allotted time, filled the prescription for pain and swelling, and went home. Not long after, I was lying down resting, and the pain came back worse than before. I called the doctor's office, and they went over my symptoms. They determined I must be allergic to one of the ingredients in what I had been given. I was instructed on what to do and told to stay off my feet until the symptoms subsided.

I was struggling with my health, and the things I had taken to relieve the pain had made it worse. I went and got a cane to help me get around. It helped a little to lean on something when standing or getting up. My steps were slower with the cane. I felt I should try a different approach. I called a chiropractor's office to see whether they could help me. I made the appointment—still trying to find a solution and not just giving up and letting it stay this way.

The chiropractor took x-rays and said he felt it was more than strained muscles or a pinched nerve. He asked me to come back for the results. I had to have some help to get to my car. He told me to see if someone could drive for me on my next appointment. My daughter, Joy, drove me to find out about my results. There was lots of activity in their office, and they put us in an examination room. When the doctor came in with another doctor, I knew they had found something. We went to the room where I could be shown my x-rays. The doctor traced where he had found an abnormality, and he said I could possibly have a fractured hip.

I was surprised at the diagnosis. He asked whether I had tripped or fallen at some point recently. Maybe bumped hard against something or perhaps even fallen out of bed. I told the doctor that I did sometimes get dizzy, but I knew to get to a lower level. I had not taken any falls. I couldn't fall out of bed because I slept on the floor.

The doctor asked whether I was doing this because of a bad back. I told him that my bed had gotten ruined in a move. I put down blankets on top of an exercise mat and then put bedding over that.

He asked how I got around in my apartment. I said, "Well, I have to crawl to the bathroom, and then I can get up. I use the cane to get around and lean on it to stand."

The doctor was shaking his head in disbelief. I asked what the treatment was for a suspected fractured hip. He said he recommended I go straight to the hospital. I asked about going to my family doctor. He told me it was best to call and see what they would want me to do.

I called my family doctor, and they said if I had x-rays to take the copies to the hospital. My coming in to them was not necessary, as they were not equipped to help with a fractured hip at their facility. The chiropractor made a disc to give to the hospital with my tests on it.

My daughter Joy took me to the hospital. She was wondering what they would do for a fractured hip. I said I knew it depended on where the bone was fractured and how bad. Joy asked how I would get around, since I lived alone. I said, "I can only do what I can do, and the rest is up to God." I told her I wasn't worried. Knowing what the problem is becomes the start of the solution.

The hospital staff was concerned about me and put me in an examination room right away. I gave them the computer disc and let them know what the chiropractor suspected was wrong. The hospital ordered some more x-rays from different angles so they would have as much information as possible. After the x-rays, they put me back in the examination room and said they would be back with their findings.

Two doctors came into the room, and we knew they had found something significant to reveal. They asked whether they could speak in front of Joy. I told them she was my daughter, and she would want to know the results. The doctor said, "You have cancer."

I said, "Okay, so what is our plan of action?"

The doctor was a bit taken back and told me I didn't seem surprised. I said, "I have had cancer come and go multiple times. We just have another diagnosis of cancer, and I am prepared to fight it."

The next questions were about who was seeing me for my cancer. I informed them I could not pay out of pocket, so my cancer doctor could not see me. There were gasps and concerns that I had not been seen for cancer in quite a while. I was told the doctor I had seen before had retired. I asked whether there was any doctor taking new patients who would take low-income patients. The doctor left the room to make some calls.

He came back with an appointment to see a cancer doctor. I thanked them for their help and said I would make sure to be there early so I could get my medical records. They said it was not necessary; the doctor would be able to acquire the records from my previous doctor.

My daughter needed to take me around because I could not drive a car. We met with the new doctor. He wanted to know whether I could stand, and then he asked to see me walk. I could stand to the count of three, and I could only take about three steps before I had to sit back down. I told the doctor it was too painful to do more. My leg had been bothering me since October of last year, and this was the beginning of March.

He listened to all the things I had done and the many thoughts of what it could be from other doctors. After hearing about my crawling to the bathroom, he said he wanted me in the hospital. The staff would start making preparations, and I was to go home and pack my things for an extended stay. They would call me later that day when it was arranged. The doctor reassured me they would do all they could to make me better.

I thanked the doctor for taking care of my case. I said, "I sort of got pushed into your patient list with no prior information." He said he had my history, and we would work together to beat cancer this time, too. I was grateful to have a doctor who was looking at all of my health issues.

My daughter took me home so I could get things packed. Joy wanted to know whether I was nervous about going into the hospital for more than three weeks. I said the doctors would be able to keep track of my progress better this way. I knew there was going to be a long list of tests and scans they would set up. If I had any trouble, I would be in the right place to get the care I needed.

I called my son, Pete, and let him know I was going to stay in the hospital for some time. Joy was going to keep him informed, and I would let him know the room number in the hospital after I got there.

Pete was anxious about how long I was staying in the hospital. I said I wasn't worried, and he should not be either. Pete said that was easy to say, but not such an easy thing for him to do. Some people have a hard time digesting news about their family member's health. They can't take too much information in, and this can be just as bad if it is too little information. Pete was one of those people where he has to have the right amount of information to absorb. Later, it proved to be too much for him—until he came to the hospital for a visit and saw me for himself.

I got the call to come back to the hospital. I got checked in, and people helped us put my things away. I got into my hospital gown and waited for the doctor. I was going to be seeing several doctors with different specialties. I had a bone biopsy to determine what type of cancer I was dealing with this time. The tests came back, and they said I didn't need surgery to remove any bone or require amputation. It was adding to and not eating away at the bones in my leg.

The tests had shown there were too many lumps to count. I was going to have radiation for fifteen days, and they only did it Monday through Friday. Few tests were done over the weekend. I had several therapy options to help relax the body and mind. I had aromatherapy and pet therapy. There was a minister who helped with soul therapy. Everyone was encouraging and hopeful of my getting better in the hospital.

Pain levels are a factor in healthcare. I was having trouble finding a comfortable way to sit or lie down. I asked whether they had air cushions to relieve the pressure points to lower the pain. Acupressure has many medicinal ways to alleviate the paths of pain. They brought in an air mattress, which they strapped to the hospital bed. No more pain meant I could sleep through the night. Being well rested helps in healing the body.

I picked "Energized" in my aromatherapy. Every time I smelled it, I felt like working harder at my recovery. With the pet therapy, all of my levels noticeably improved. The doctor even mentioned he could tell what days I'd had a visit from the pets. I told him they see the person first and the illness second. Animals can sense many things. They have an uncanny knack for wanting to make things better for you and know how to do it.

I followed the hospital procedures. During my stay, it was discovered I have lymphedema when an IV or a blood pressure cuff is used on my right side. The lymphedema was put on my charts as an adverse reaction, and I had therapy to remove the excess fluids. I am grateful this happened in a hospital and people knew what to do. I am watchful over my health issues, and I can help in keeping me healthy.

I had many people come to see me in the hospital. My visitors were amazed at my progress. I had learned to use a walker. I had a nurse go with me to go around the hospital ward. At first, I could not go too far before needing to turn around. But I was determined to be mobile. I was surpassing all of the goals they set for me.

My visitors had a written log they could see of what I had done that day. I told them God wants us to exceed in all we do. If reaching my goal was the best I could do, then God would be happy. If I could surpass the goal, then everyone knew I was following the higher instruction of God.

When you are weak, God brings strength. When you are sick, God brings peace to a world where worry is prevalent. Finding peace with God helps you to heal the body. You must seek God first to find Him. If you know God, you can have God in your life. It is a choice God allows each of us to make.

As I was nearing the end of my radiation treatment. The doctor came by to let me know I was progressing beyond expectations. I would have therapists coming to my house to help with strengthening exercises. My doctor asked how I felt about leaving the hospital and being on my own.

I said, "God has made the lame to walk and the blind to see. I know because He has done this for me." I told him God would still be watching over me. The doctor agreed I'd had help in my recovery, as he had seen it firsthand.

The doctor said I was going to receive a walker to use in my home. He was also ordering a hospital bed to be delivered to my home when I was discharged. I could take the air mattress that I had been using at the hospital. I told the doctor I was so grateful for all the care and concern given to me. The doctor said I was doing everything asked of me and still striving to do more. I would have follow-up visits with the doctor. I had new medicine I had been taking while in the hospital, and I would continue with when I was released.

The doctor asked whether I had any questions or concerns. I asked about what activities I could do. The doctor said I was not to lift anything over five pounds. I was to use my discretion about how long to walk, stand, or sit. The therapists would go over what to look for in warning signs that I was doing too much or too soon. I told the doctor I would be careful. I said I was going to keep improving when I got home. The doctor agreed I should keep positive about my continuing recovery from this latest bout with cancer.

Before I left the hospital, I had the names and numbers of people to call and several appointments made for follow-ups. I had an initial assessment scheduled to see what I could do on my own around the house. Joy was taking me home and said she had some concerns about what I could do on my own. I had been in the hospital for twenty-four days, and people were around all the time. Joy said she could not stay with me at my place and go to work as well. I told Joy I was going to figure it all out. I would do what I could and ask for help when needed. Joy said she had a feeling I would find out very quickly what I could not do without help.

Joy got me back home, and we called the people about bringing the hospital bed. They informed me it would be tomorrow before they got to me. They had more deliveries than usual and had gotten behind. Joy asked whether I was going to go back to sleeping on the floor. I said I would use the twin sized mattress she'd slept on while she was looking after my home. I would use the cane to get down and up from it. Joy asked about moving things out of the way. I told her I only had so much space, and we would have to stack things up. We made a pathway for the walker so I could use it when I needed more support than a cane.

Joy was reluctant to leave me alone. I told her I had to start learning to do things on my own again. It might have to be modified to accommodate what I was able to do now. I just had to try and see. Joy asked what I was going to do first. I said I was tired, and I wanted to get some sleep. Joy helped me make my makeshift bed. She made sure I was able to use the cane to get on and off the mattress. I had to show her I could get in and out of the bathroom on my own. Joy was satisfied I was able to move about without any issues. I left nightlights on to help me to see if I had to get up in the night. Joy left, and I went to sleep tired but happy to be home.

The next day, I found that simple tasks I had taken for granted as every day and uneventful had become unwieldly and awkward. My restrictions had me confused as how to do my laundry. I could not lift the basket or the detergent with a five-pound limit. I went to go see whether I could borrow some rope or something I could drag to the laundry room. One of the tenants came back with a wheeled walker with a basket and a seat on it. He said it was old, he did not need it anymore, and I could have it. I was excited and said, "Thank you so much, it is perfect."

He helped adjust the height, so I was not bending over so much. Then he got an old rag and cleaned off the dust. He said he was glad somebody could get some use out of it. He helped me move it into my apartment, and I thanked him again for such a wonderful gift.

Now I was truly able to get things done. It was not the same as before, but I felt the independence had uplifted my spirit. Each task had to be looked at and seen from a different perspective. "What can I do to make this work?" was the question I asked myself throughout the day.

I called about the hospital bed, and the man said he was short staffed again. It would be Sunday afternoon now before he would have it delivered. I thanked him for letting me know and asked whether he had an estimated time. He said he would call at noon, and he would have a better idea then.

On Sunday I got the call I had been waiting for about the hospital bed. He had a question for me. He was close to my home. His crew was taking their lunch. Did I want the bed today or could I wait until Monday? I said I would really like the bed today. He said he would skip his lunch and bring the bed over. I gave him the address again and waited. He showed up and said it would take several trips to bring the parts into the hallway outside my door.

I innocently asked whether it would take long to put together after the area was cleared. He stopped and said he didn't do any of the lifting—that is what his crew did. He was just dropping off. I asked whether he could put it together. He said, "You would have to move everything out of the way for me." Otherwise, I would be putting the bed together myself.

I knew I could push things, but lifting would have to be creative. This man was not going to budge on what he was willing to do. He had skipped his lunch and left his crew to get the parts to me. I said, "I will get the place cleared for you, and you can put it together."

He agreed and told me I had to be quick about it since he had to get back to his crew.

Obstacles are things in your way. They can be physical or mental. I had to think of only moving everything out of the way in the space of time I was given. He had two more trips, and I had to be done with moving. I used my cane in ways it was never intended to be used. A lever is a powerful tool. It allows you to lift things easier. My cane became a lever. I became a mover of bigger things than me. The last thing to move was the mattress. I got it on its side and held it in place.

The man poked his head in the door and asked whether I had it ready for him. I said, "Everything is out of your way." He moved the parts inside and grabbed his tools. It was an electric hospital bed, and he made sure it reached the outlet. In fifteen minutes, I had a bed. He had to get back to his crew. I thanked him for putting the bed together for me as he went out the door.

I had been holding the mattress the whole time. I now had another dilemma. How do I get the mattress out of the way? I had a pathway, and I could get it into another room now that I was not time constrained. A mattress does not like being on its side, and it moves to get back to its preferred and designed position. I used toes, hips, and arms to keep it upright and slowly pulled it to another room. I eased the mattress down. I thought God had given me strength I did not have, and He gave me a mind to figure out the way. As I was thanking God for His help, I realized it was what I needed to do in therapy as well. God was showing me the way.

I was in a place of certain health limitations for now. Work within the framework given. Then find a way to get where you want to be. I wanted my goal of being able to walk again without a walker or a cane. I was going to exceed expectations and go beyond what was not even considered possible.

My therapy assessment started on Monday. I had to go through and show what I could do on my own. It was marked off as a task completed successfully. Next came what I needed assistance with and what strengthening and stretching exercises would be utilized to get ready for my personalized regimen. They asked what my energy level was like. I said I was ready to start the exercise program.

I was shown each exercise and the proper way to do it. I had to show I could do it and then do so many and count my way of holding each one. At the end of the session, I was given a goal to do every day until they returned.

I had assessments all week. If I needed anything, I had a list of people to call. My goals were written down. I was given exercise sheets that went step by step on how to do them, how many, and how long to hold the count. I made sure I did the exercises properly and tried to do a little more each time. I did them throughout the day. I was determined to do my very best.

I noticed during certain exercises that I was having difficulty. I pointed it out to my therapist. She asked me what I thought. I said, "My spine is not straight." I wanted to know whether there were exercises to straighten my spine. She said we could try one and see whether it helped any. She told me what to do and how long to hold it. She said, "Now, slowly try and see what happens when you stand up."

It worked. I didn't feel the muscles pulling anymore. We tried one of the exercises I had trouble doing, and I could do it with ease. After that, I just kept adding different exercises and eliminating the ones I no longer needed.

Slowly and surely, I needed less and less physical therapy. All of my progress was documented and sent to the cancer doctor. I had set a goal for myself when I saw the doctor for my first follow-up. I wanted to be less dependent on the walker. I finished all the physical therapy ahead of schedule. I knew this would be astonishing news by itself, but I wanted to be even further in my progress. I kept working at it, and gradually I could walk around with the cane in my home more and use the walker less. When I went for my cancer doctor appointment, I had to use the walker because of how big the place was, and I didn't want to overtax myself.

The doctor said I had gotten to be quite the expert getting around with my walker. I told him I had gotten further in my progress than he realized. I showed him I could use the cane and walk alone for short distances. I could stand for a longer length of time. I told him I was going to be working hard to get even stronger. The doctor was impressed at how well I was doing. He asked how I felt and what my pain level was. I said, "I am down to a one or two pain level. Next time, I will not have any pain, and I will be stronger."

The next appointment I came in with my cane and no walker needed except for help in carrying heavy items. My pain was gone, and I told the doctor I would keep improving.

My next appointment, I came with no cane. The doctor was looking for it, and I said, "I don't need it." I stood up and said, "I also can walk backwards." I showed him, and then I said, "I can dance," and took some steps. I said, "If you like, I can run for you, too."

The doctor said it was amazing progress. He could hardly believe this was the same person who'd had to crawl to get around in her home before. He said I should be very proud of what I had accomplished.

I told the doctor, "I can do nothing without God." I had been shown what to do, and the doctor had given me goals and medicine, which helped me to improve. I said, "I could have stopped there, but God has plans for me. I certainly didn't want to let God down." I told the doctor I was writing a book about my life. God wanted me to help people. I said, "I think my story could be an encouragement for others." The doctor agreed and said my faith in God was a testament in itself. Then I added my cancer journey to it. He said it was showing body, mind, and soul working together to heal.

God knows what we need before we do. I was making progress. I was slower than I was before in walking. God had a plan to kick it up a notch. People go to a level they are comfortable with and then level off. God knew I needed incentive to go further and faster.

My daughter, Joy, called me and said there was an urgent need, and she wanted my help. Joy said a puppy needed a home, and she couldn't have pets where she lived. Pets were allowed where I lived. I said it was not something I had thought about for a long time. Joy said, "Please. You can help people, so why not a puppy?"

Joy knew I loved animals. I said, first of all, I would have to get permission. I would have to physically be able to do it. Joy said she would help me to find out whether it was possible. Joy would work with me to see what the doctor said I would physically need help with. I agreed to look into doing it.

Everyone worked to make it happen. My cancer doctor thought it was a fantastic idea and faxed the information needed to my apartment manager. It was deemed I needed a support animal to help aid in my recovery. My daughter signed papers that she would be responsible to care for the puppy if I needed to go to the hospital or if I became incapacitated or died. Joy would also help with making sure the dog received all her well visits and shots.

Joy brought a ten-week-old puppy with her food and dishes. You could hold the puppy in your two hands. Joy told me she was a Chihuahua. She was a little shy at first, but soon she was off exploring her new home. We decided to call her Pinky, since she'd come to help a breast cancer survivor.

Pinky has a pink baby blanket she sleeps with to keep her warm. We found out our little addition definitely likes to snuggle. I made a bed for her, and she kept trying to find me. I put her in my lap, and she curled up and went to sleep.

When we took Pinky to the veterinarian for her shots, I found out she was not a purebred dog. The veterinarian asked if it made a difference. I said, "I am just glad she is healthy." I asked what kind of dog Pinky was, and the vet said she is a Chiweenie, a cross between a Chihuahua and a Dachshund. Pinky got a clean bill of health, and that is what counts.

Pinky got acclimated to her new home, and soon she was meeting different people and dogs. It was very important to have her well socialized to be a happy and healthy dog. Pinky loves walks, and I soon found out why God sent her to me. Pinky runs like a Husky.

She drives forward with her front paws, and her back legs are moving together to pull. God sent me full circle, and my walks were no longer slow. I had to go at a much faster pace to keep up with Pinky.

When I went back to the cancer doctor for my checkup, he told me how fast I was walking was surprising. I told him Pinky needed to be walked often, and it was always at a rapid pace. I asked the doctor whether I was doing okay. He said if we both bowed down flat to the floor in thanks to God for what He has done, it wouldn't begin to be enough. My doctor said I had gone on to be more than a miracle; I was beyond a miracle.

I said, "It is God who has kept me here. God has a purpose for me and is making sure I am ready to get it done. I told the doctor we were a team. With God's help, I was still here and doing better than anyone thought possible.

If you honor God in faith, God will honor your faith. God has put me on the path of His purpose for me. I am going forward with what God has called me to do.

I know God has more plans for me as I continue to follow Him. I have made mistakes along the way. I learned from them and kept going forward. I have shared my past so that you may understand where I am in my present. My future is held in God's hands. All along I have known my time here is limited. God has kept me here to share the things that He wants you most to know. God is real; God is here. He has been right beside me through everything. The world sees negative things, but God makes things positive.

Have you been looking for something in this life to fulfill you and to make your life one that has meaning? Then know this: what you search for has been put into every human being. You are looking for God, and He is right here, right now, waiting for you to discover Him. While He has been writing my life story—He has been writing yours as well.

BIO

Merrily Opal Pearl is an author, cancer survivor, and an inspirational speaker who passionately shares about her relationship with God and His transformative impact on her life. Merrily truly believes that God makes us bigger than ourselves with the gifts He gives us. "Nothing is by chance—everything is God's plan," she writes. "God looks for people who are willing and available to do what others are not."

Merrily has become a bold and fearless person—not of her own accord but because God challenged her to be, do, and think differently than everyone else.

www.ingramcontent.com/pod-product-compliance
Lightning Source LLC
Chambersburg PA
CBHW051957290426
44110CB00015B/2283